Food *for* Life

Acknowledgments

We would like to thank Jane Johnstone, Gemma Bircher and the renal dietetic team at Leicester General Hospital for their input with this book.

Published by Baxter Healthcare Renal Division,
Wallingford Road, Compton, Newbury, Berkshire, UK
Telephone 01635 206000

ISBN 0-9528823-1-0

Produced for Baxter Healthcare by Wavelength PR
Designed by Quadrant Communications Ltd
Photography by Peter Dawes
Winchester, UK

December 1998

Contents

Foreword

Why have a cookery book for dialysis patients? Having been involved in dialysis for the past seven years, five of which have been concerned with nutrition in end stage renal failure patients, I have become concerned about the dietary limitations for those on dialysis.

Being a bit of a 'foodie' I put myself in the position of the patients we treat and wondered how I would feel about the limitations imposed on what I could and could not eat. There are many recipe books available for dialysis patients, but these mostly contain variations of standard English food. This made me think that there must be a way of producing interesting food which complies with dietary restrictions, but at the same time was imaginative and could be eaten quite happily by the rest of the family and friends.

With this in mind I contacted the Chef's Association to investigate whether I could find a chef to work with on this project. This is where fate played a hand. Having been given the number by Good Food Magazine I contacted who I thought was the secretary of the Association. Instead Lawrence Keogh, a top London chef, answered the phone.

Having briefly explained to him what I was trying to do he said that he would be interested in helping with the project as it transpired that he was a pre-dialysis patient at a unit in London.

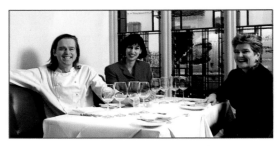

From left to right: Lawrence Keogh, Rashmi Soni and Jane Leonard

A renal dietitian I had been working with for some time on other projects, Rashmi Soni, also agreed to give us her guidance and expertise. This has ensured that the recipes take into account the widely differing needs of renal patients. The result of this collaboration is this book which I hope you will enjoy and that it will inspire you to create your own 'renal conscious' recipes.

Janet Leonard.

Jane Leonard
Baxter Healthcare

3

" When you are diagnosed with kidney failure, quite simply your life changes fundamentally. Suddenly you and your family are faced with a new lifestyle which can be extremely difficult and challenging to cope with. Limitations to what you can eat and drink are particularly frustrating with many favourite foods suddenly out of bounds and trips to restaurants a nightmare. Even entertaining family and friends can be stressful trying to think of new and interesting recipes which all can eat and enjoy.

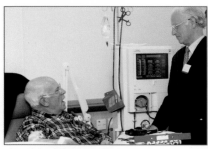

Lord Norrie meeting a patient.

4

That is why I think this recipe book is so refreshing. Written by a top London chef, himself a dialysis patient, it contains beautifully created recipes which are ideal for special occasions. I am delighted that Baxter Healthcare, who have produced this book, have kindly donated all proceeds from its sale to the National Kidney Federation, the national charity run by kidney patients for the benefits of kidney patients. "

Norrie

Lord Norrie
President, National Kidney Federation

Introduction

It is hoped that this cookery book will inspire you to try out different recipes and ingredients you may not normally eat. It is not so much an everyday cook book but one that can be used for special occasions as the nutritional values may be higher than normal.

By listing the nutritional analysis for each recipe, you will be able to see exactly what it contains and use this information to plan your menu accordingly. For example, if you are planning a high potassium main meal then you should make sure that the starter and dessert is low in potassium and that any vegetable accompaniments are also low (see Quick Guide section for low potassium vegetable suggestions).

You should also be aware of other meals you are eating during the day to make sure that your total daily nutritional intake is not exceeded. To help you, a summary of the nutritional values for all recipes is included in the Quick Guide section together with suggested menu plans. We have also added a herb and spice reference guide should you wish to experiment with some of these recipes but safely keep within the correct nutritional values.

In the portion guide for each recipe we have either given the exact portion amount or how many the dish should be divided into. It is important to remember that the nutritional analysis is based on the portion or serving size and does not include any accompaniments.

Remember that not all of these recipes may be suitable for you so be sure to keep within your dietitian's guidelines. Be aware that all fluid based recipes must be within your fluid or milk allowance. If in doubt, talk to your renal dietitian.

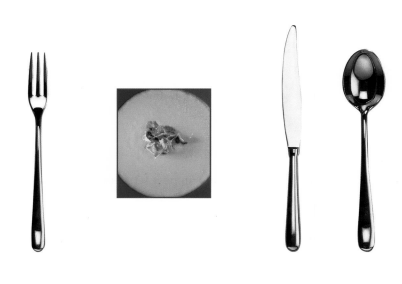

Starters

Preparation time 20 minutes
Cooking time 45 minutes

Nutritional Content:
Energy 38 Kcal, 160 kJ
Protein 0.41 g
Fat 2.32 g
Sodium 3.90 mmol
Potassium 1.42 mmol
Phosphorus 0.32 mmol

EQUIPMENT

Thick bottomed saucepan
with a lid.

Liquidiser or hand blender.

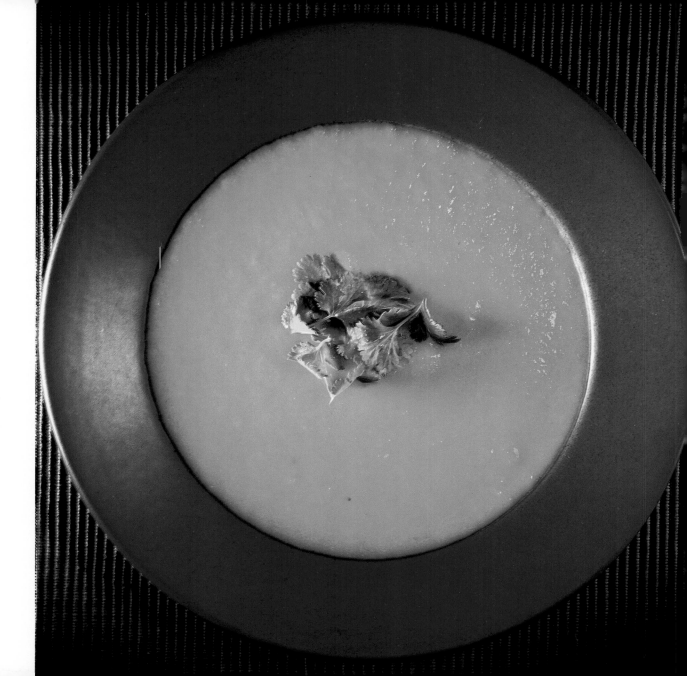

Carrot and Coriander Soup

Soup makes an easy hot starter for a dinner party as it can be made in advance and then reheated.

Alternatively it will make a filling snack, and this recipe could not be easier.

It can also be made and frozen in serving sized portions and then reheated and garnished

with the coriander leaves just before serving.

INGREDIENTS

Carrots	1¼ lb/570g chopped
Onions	2½ oz/70g chopped
Bay Leaves	2
Whole Peppercorns	3
Leeks	2½ oz/70g chopped
Salt	pinch/2g
Fresh Pepper	pinch/2g
Sugar	1½ oz/45g
Ginger	½ oz/15g grated
Nutmeg	½ oz/15g grated
Butter	1½ oz/45g
Coriander Leaves	10
Water	2 pints/1.2 litre
Coriander Seeds	6

1 Place all ingredients, except the water and coriander leaves in a thick bottomed pan. Cover with lid and cook without liquid until half cooked stirring occasionally to prevent the mixture catching on the bottom of the pan.

2 Add water and bring to the boil, reduce heat to simmer for approximately 30-45 minutes.

3 Remove soup from heat and blend either in a liquidiser or using a hand held blender until smooth. Adjust seasoning and consistency if needed.

4 To serve, sprinkle ground coriander over the surface.

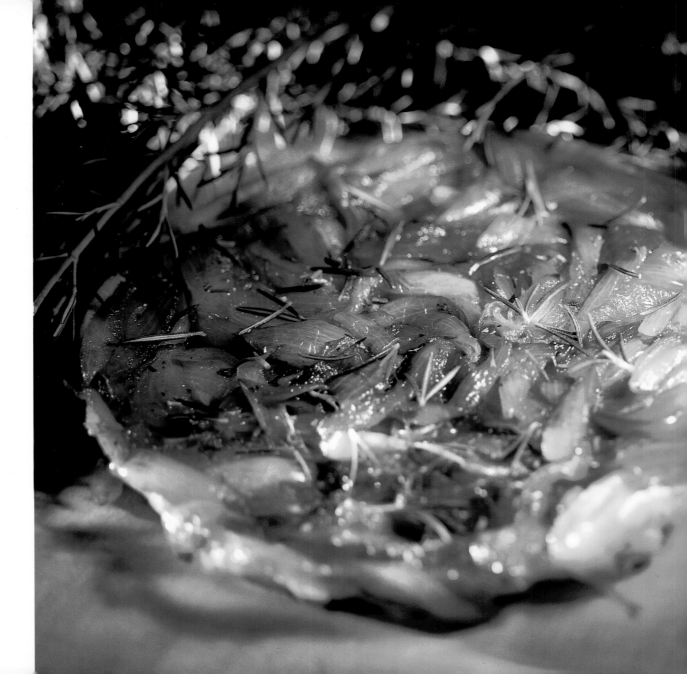

Preparation time 20 minutes
Cooking time 15-20 minutes

Nutritional Content:
Energy 343 Kcal, 1426 kJ
Protein 4.15 g
Fat 23.67 g
Sodium 11.77 mmol
Potassium 4.15 mmol
Phosphorus 1.78 mmol

EQUIPMENT

Frying pan (approximately
8 inches or 20cm) that can go
into the oven.

Large plate that is wider than
the frying pan.

Onion and Rosemary Tart Tatin

This is a dish which always looks good and will make an impressive first course without spending hours in the kitchen. To make it easy to prepare, use ready prepared puff pastry.

INGREDIENTS

Red and White Onions	1¼ lb/570g sliced thickly root on
Unsalted Butter	4 oz/110g
Rosemary, lightly chopped	8 sprigs
Ground Pepper	pinch/2g
Sugar	1 oz/28g
Puff Pastry	1 lb/450g

1 Fry onions in a pan that can go in the oven (approximately 8 inches or 20cm), until deep golden brown.

2 Add rosemary, sugar and pepper, then take off the heat.

3 Roll out puff pastry, so that it can cover pan, let it rest for 10 minutes then lay puff pastry over onions like a lid. Then place pan in oven and cook for approximately 15-20 minutes until puff pastry has risen and is golden brown.

4 Have a large plate that is wider than the surface area of the pan ready.

5 When you have removed the tart from the oven let it stand for a couple of minutes to cool then place the plate on top of the onion tart and turn over very quickly.

6 The onion tart is now ready to serve.

Preparation time 15 minutes
Cooking time 45 minutes

Nutritional Content:
Energy 30 Kcal, 126 kJ
Protein 1.24 g
Fat 1.17 g
Sodium 1.61 mmol
Potassium 5.22 mmol
Phosphorus 0.72 mmol

EQUIPMENT

Thick bottomed saucepan
with a lid.

Liquidiser or hand blender.

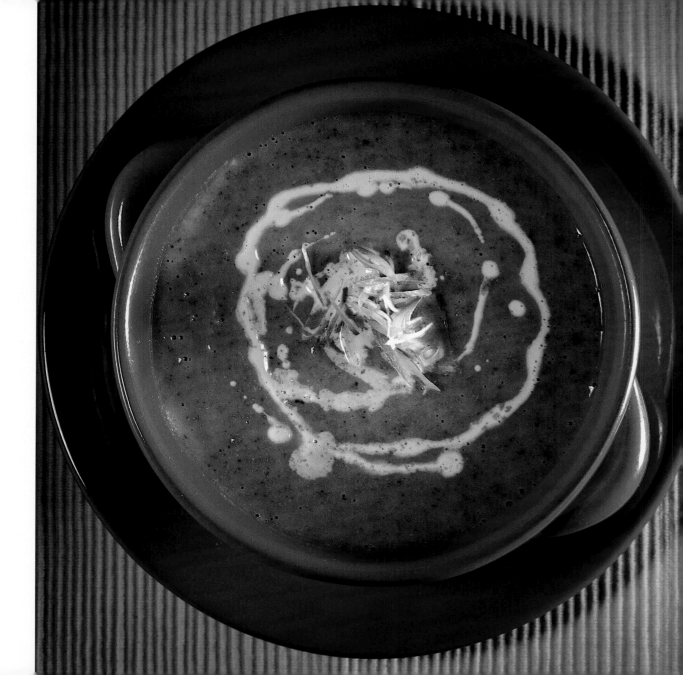

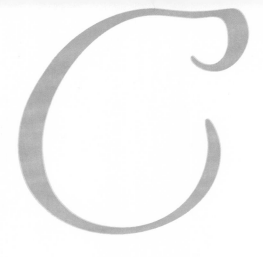

Cream of Courgette and Cumin Soup

– SERVES 6 –
– PORTION SIZE 5½ floz/160ml –

INGREDIENTS

Courgette	2 lb 3 oz/1kg
Leek	2 oz/55g
Onion	3 oz/85g
Shallots	2 oz/55g
Lemon Thyme	pinch/2g
Cumin	2 oz/55g
Bay Leaves	2
Whole Peppercorns	3
Olive Oil	4 tsp/20ml
Water	1¾ pint/1 litre
Salt	pinch/2g
Fresh Black Pepper	pinch/2g
Sugar	1 oz/28g
Cream	2 tsp/10ml

1 Using a thick bottomed saucepan place the oil in the pan and heat.

2 Roughly cut courgettes, leeks, onion, shallots and add to pan along with thyme, cumin, bay leaves, peppercorns.

3 Cook in oil, stirring all the time, until all ingredients have wilted.

4 Add water to the pan, bring the liquid to the boil and then reduce the heat to a slight simmer for approximately 30-40 minutes.

5 Take the saucepan off the heat and with a liquidiser or blender, blend the soup until smooth.

6 Once the soup is smooth add the salt, pepper, sugar and cream to your taste.

15

Preparation time 20 minutes
Cooking time 45 minutes

Nutritional Content:
Energy 48 Kcal, 189 kJ
Protein 1.59 g
Fat 2.66 g
Sodium 8.96 mmol
Potassium 5.81 mmol
Phosphorus 1.14 mmol

EQUIPMENT

Thick bottomed saucepan
with a lid.

Liquidiser or hand blender.

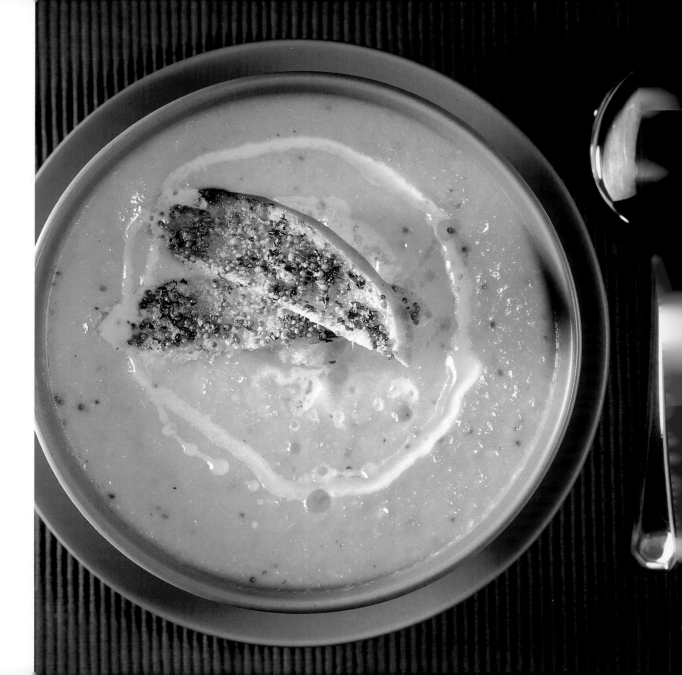

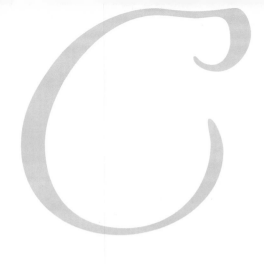

Cream of Cauliflower and Mustard Soup

− SERVES 6 −
− PORTION SIZE 5½ floz/160ml −

INGREDIENTS

Cauliflower	2 lb 3 oz/1kg in florets
Onion	3 oz/85g chopped
Celery	3 oz/85g chopped
Leek	3 oz/85g chopped
Garlic	2 cloves crushed
Potato	5 oz/140g chopped
Grain Mustard	1 oz/28g
Dijon Mustard	1 oz/28g
Butter (unsalted)	2 oz/55g
Bay Leaves	2
Whole Peppercorns	3
Salt	pinch/2g
Sugar	½ oz/15g
Water	2 pint/1.2 litre

For the Garnish

Cauliflower Florets	5 pieces/50g
Ciabatta Bread	3 slices/75g
Parsley	½ oz/15g
Grain Mustard	½ oz/15g
Olive Oil	1 tbsp/15ml

1 Melt butter in a thick bottomed pan and then add all the ingredients except the water.

2 Sweat all the ingredients in the pan until half cooked, then add the water and bring to the boil, once boiled turn the heat down and simmer for approximately 30-40 minutes.

3 Remove the pan from the stove and with a liquidiser or blender, blend the soup until smooth, adjust the taste with mustard and sugar if need be.

4 **Garnish:** Blanch the florets in boiling water for approximately 5 minutes, then refresh in cold water. Mix the mustard, parsley and oil together until bound. Spread mustard mix smoothly over bread and grill until crunchy, then cut into croutons.

5 **To Serve:** Reheat the soup, then pour into the serving bowl, place the cauliflower florets into the middle of the soup with the croutons on top.

Preparation time 25 minutes
Cooking time 8-10 minutes

Nutritional Content:
Energy 255 Kcal, 1228 kJ
Protein 10.94 g
Fat 16.18 g
Sodium 7.05 mmol
Potassium 5.85 mmol
Phosphorus 3.71 mmol

EQUIPMENT

Wok or large frying pan.

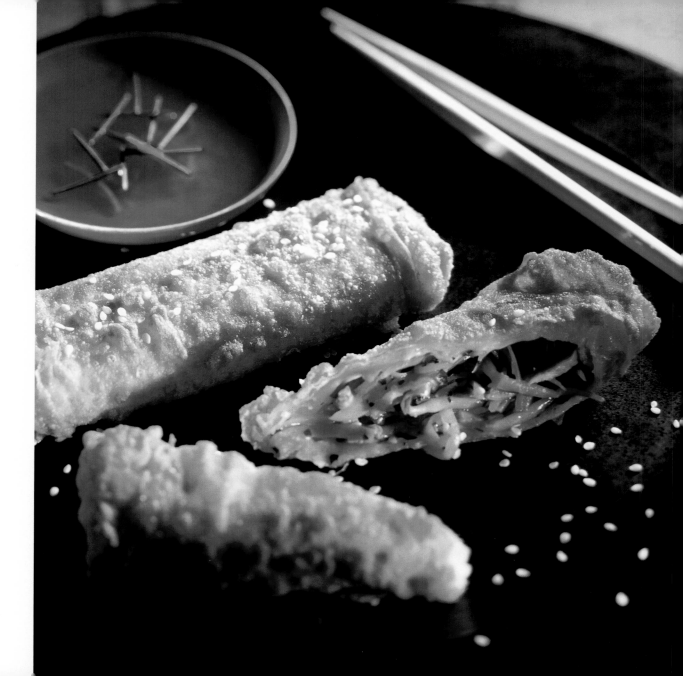

Chicken Spring Rolls

An easy to make starter that tastes as though it has come right out of a Chinese kitchen. Because it can be prepared ahead it minimises last minute preparation and leaves you time to relax before your meal.

INGREDIENTS

Filo Pastry	2 sheets
Beansprouts	6 oz / 170g
Carrots	3 oz / 85g thin strips
Spring Onions	1½ oz / 45g chopped
Garlic	2 cloves
Root Ginger	1 tsp chopped
Fresh Mint	1 tsp
Coriander	1 tsp
Chicken	8 oz / 225g skin removed
Oil	3 tsp / 15ml
Sesame Oil	2 drops / 1ml
Black Pepper	pinch / 2g freshly milled
Cornflour	4 tsp
Egg White	1
Light Soy Sauce	1 floz / 30ml
Olive Oil for brushing	1 tbsp / 15ml

1 Cut chicken into fine strips and fry in hot wok with a little oil flavoured with sesame oil.

2 Add the chopped ginger, garlic and stir. Toss in carrots and beansprouts and cook for a few minutes. Season with pepper.

3 Take off heat and stir in mint and coriander and allow to cool.

4 Spread filo pastry out in a large square - two sheets only. Cut strips length wise, approximately 6 inches (15cm) across.

5 Place some of the filling at one end, leaving ½ inch either side of the filling.

6 Fold the outside into the middle and roll around approximately twice. Seal with lightly beaten egg white and place onto a cloth that has been sprinkled with cornflour.

7 Keep in the fridge until needed. Brush with oil and bake at 220°C, 425°F, Gas Mark 7 for 8-10 minutes.

8 Serve as a starter with the Asian Spring Roll dipping sauce on page 20.

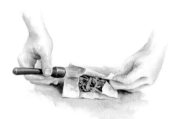

Rolling a Spring Roll.

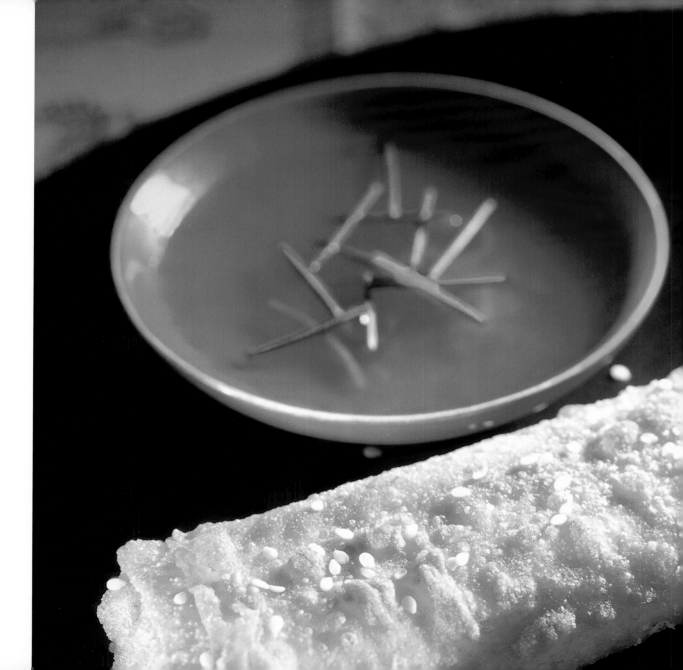

Preparation time 5 minutes
Cooking time 15 minutes

Nutritional Content:
Energy 68 Kcal, 291 kJ
Protein 0.11 g
Fat 0.02 g
Sodium 0.02 mmol
Potassium 0.53 mmol
Phosphorus 0.07 mmol

Asian Spring Roll Dipping Sauce

This sauce makes an ideal accompaniment to the Chicken Spring Rolls on page 18.
It can be kept in a sealed container in the fridge for 2-3 weeks
and to add extra flavour can also be used to coat meat prior to grilling.

INGREDIENTS

Ingredient	Amount
Hot Water	9 floz / 255ml
Sugar	4 oz / 110g
Red Chilli	½ / 5g
Coriander Leaves	2-3 / 5g
Garlic	1 clove
Root Ginger	½ oz / 15g
Fresh Lime Juice	½ tbsp / 10mls

1 Dissolve the sugar in the water.

2 Finely chop the chilli, coriander, garlic and ginger, then add to sugar and water.

3 Bring this mixture to the boil, then simmer for 5 minutes to let flavours infuse.

4 Once the sauce has infused for 5 minutes take it off the heat and add the lime juice to taste.

5 Serve as an accompaniment to Chicken Spring Rolls.

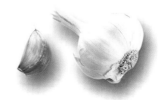

Preparation time 15 minutes
Cooking time 10-15 minutes

Nutritional Content:
Energy 731 Kcal, 3041 kJ
Protein 22.00 g
Fat 69.00 g
Sodium 3.00 mmol
Potassium 15.00 mmol
Phosphorus 10.00 mmol

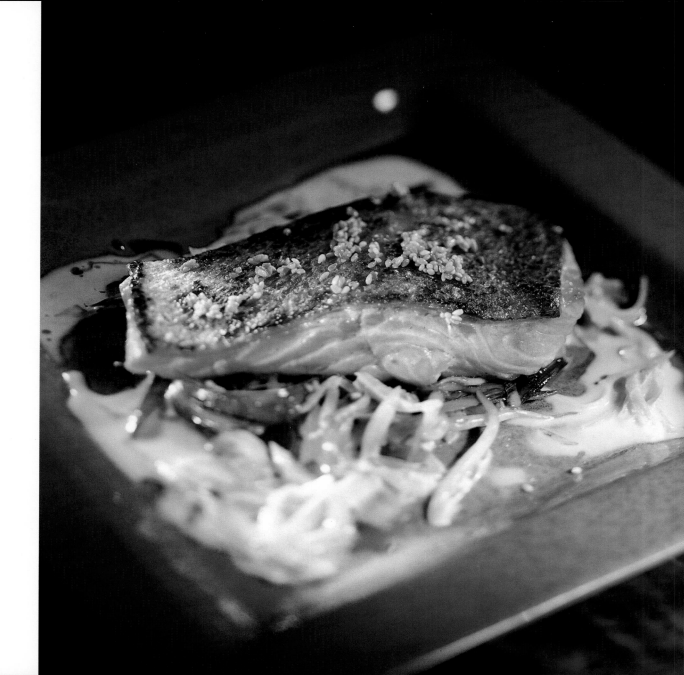

Pan Fried Salmon with a Ginger and Basil Butter Sauce

— SERVES 2 —

This makes an appetising starter and because of its richness it can be followed by a simple main course; for example pasta with a tarragon sauce or grilled white meat.

INGREDIENTS

Sesame Oil	$1/2$ tsp / 2.5ml
Salmon Steak Fillets	6 oz / 170g
Black Pepper	pinch / 2g
Mange Tout/Snow Peas	$1^1/2$ oz / 45g
Beansprouts	$1^1/2$ oz / 45g
Spring Onions	$1^1/2$ oz / 45g
Shallots	2 oz / 55g sliced
Root Ginger	$1/2$ oz / 15g cut into fine strips
Rice Wine Vinegar	4 tbsp / 60ml
Double Cream	3 floz / 90ml
Unsalted Butter	3 oz / 85g
Sesame Seeds	large pinch / 4g

1 Cut the mange tout/snow peas and spring onions into long strips and sweat in a hot pan, add beansprouts and cracked pepper.

2 To make the butter sauce, place sliced shallots, ginger and vinegar into pan and reduce by $3/4$, add cream and reduce by $1/2$, whisk in butter piece by piece continually whisking until all added.

3 Bring sauce to the boil, then take off and keep warm.

4 Roast sesame seeds under hot grill, taking care they do not burn.

5 Season salmon steak with cracked black pepper, heat oil in pan and seal salmon, skin side down first.

6 **To serve:** Place green vegetables on plate, then the salmon steak on top, pour the sauce around the plate and sprinkle the roasted sesame seeds over the top.

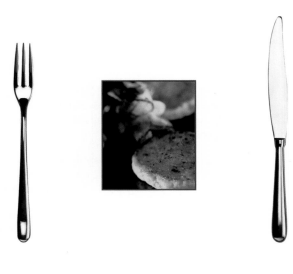

Main Courses

Preparation time 25 minutes
Cooking time 5 minutes

Nutritional Content:
Energy 123 Kcal, 516 kJ
Protein 15.33 g
Fat 6.80 g
Sodium 15.22 mmol
Potassium 8.44 mmol
Phosphorus 5.92 mmol

VARIATIONS

For a cheaper version use any white
fish that is boned and skinned.

EQUIPMENT

Blender.

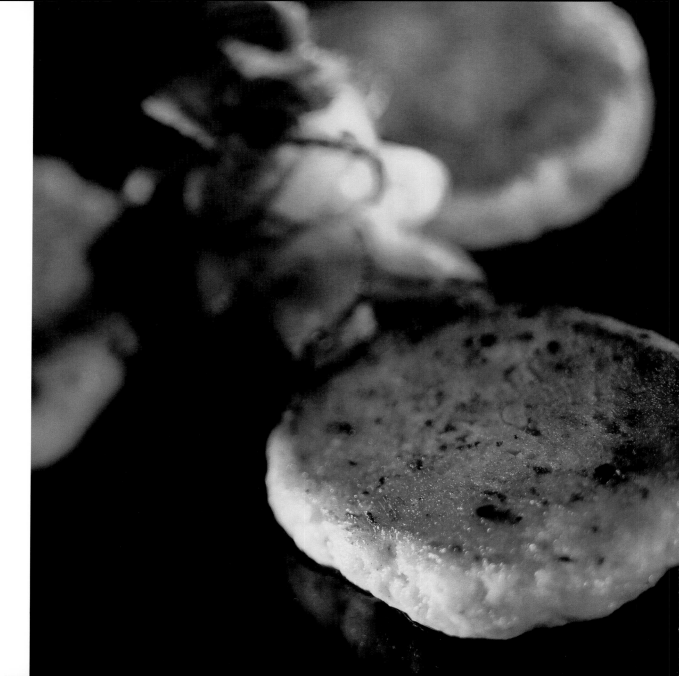

Thai Fish Cakes

You can forget the fish cakes of your school dinner days, these fish cakes are delicious and easy to make.

Serve them with plain boiled rice or some Fragrant Thai Rice that is now readily available in the supermarkets.

Depending on your potassium needs it can be accompanied either by the Thai Cucumber Salad on page 28

or an alternative low potassium vegetable.

INGREDIENTS

Salmon	4 oz/110g filleted and skinned
Cod	8 oz/225g filleted and skinned
Sesame Oil	1/2 tsp/2.5ml
Garlic	1 tbsp
Root Ginger	1 tbsp
Red Chilli (small)	1/2
Soy Sauce	1 tsp/5ml
Lemon Grass	1/2 oz/15g
Salt	pinch/2g
Pepper	pinch/2g
Lime Juice	2 tsp/10ml
Sunflower Oil for cooking	2 tsp/10ml

1 Blend all ingredients in a blender until bound together and smooth.

2 Mould into 12 small balls.

3 Heat pan on stove and cook the cakes for 5 minutes each side, flattening them down to 1 inch (2.5cm) thick while cooking.

4 Serve immediately garnished with flat leaf parsley.

Preparation time 30 minutes

Nutritional Content:
Energy 33 Kcal, 142 kJ
Protein 0.72 g
Fat 0.10 g
Sodium 0.47 mmol
Potassium 3.40 mmol
Phosphorus 1.22 mmol

EQUIPMENT

A jar with a tight fitting lid.

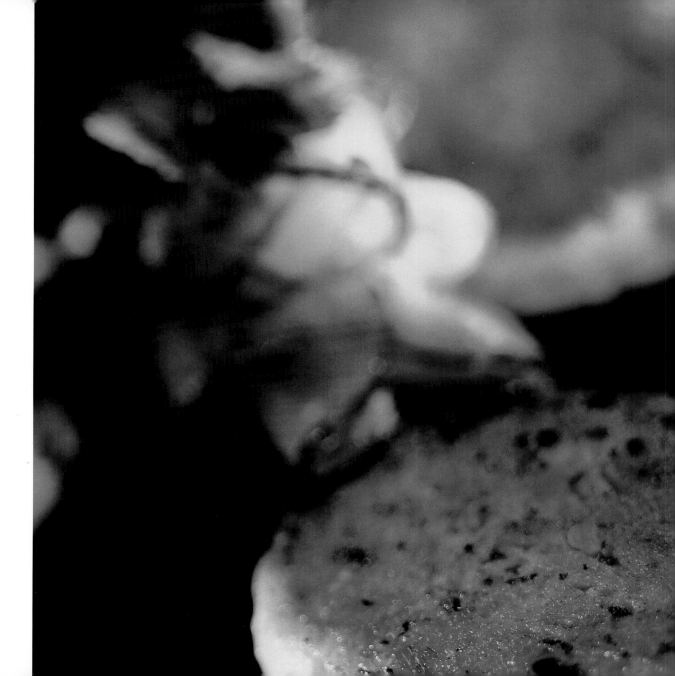

Thai Cucumber Salad

— SERVES 6 —

A great accompaniment to the Thai Fish Cakes on page 26.

INGREDIENTS

Rice or White Wine Vinegar	5 floz/150ml
Brown Sugar	2 tbsp/40g firmly packed
Cucumbers	8 oz/225g cut into $^1/_4$ inch slices
Shallots	4 thinly sliced
Chilli Pepper Flakes	$^1/_4$ tsp
Cilantro or Parsley	1 tbsp chopped

1 Combine vinegar, sugar, salt and pepper to taste, in a jar with a tight fitting lid.

2 Shake vigorously until the sugar has dissolved. Combine with remaining ingredients in a bowl.

3 Toss and marinate for at least 30 minutes before serving.

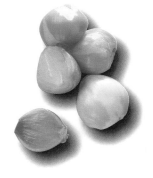

Preparation time 1 hour
Cooking time 30-40 minutes

Nutritional Content:
Energy 929 Kcal, 3860 kJ
Protein 10.10 g
Fat 73.36 g
Sodium 54.49 mmol
Potassium 11.69 mmol
Phosphorus 5.65 mmol

EQUIPMENT

Thick bottomed saucepan.

4 inch or 10cm round bowl.

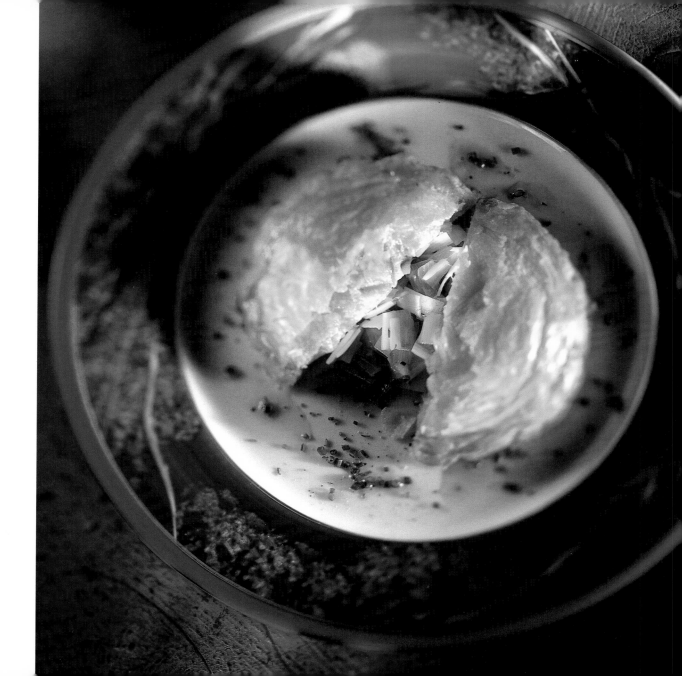

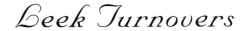

Leek Turnovers

— SERVES 4 —
— PORTION SIZE 7oz/200g —

These Turnovers make a good picnic alternative to sandwiches.

INGREDIENTS

Butter	4 oz/110g
Leek	1 lb/450g sliced
White Pepper	large pinch/4g
Salt	pinch/2g
Chives	½ bunch chopped
Puff Pastry	1 lb/450g
Egg Yolk	1

1 Melt butter in thick bottomed pan, add leeks and cook without colouring for approximately 20-30 minutes, stirring regularly. Once cooked take off the heat, season with pepper and salt. Add chives and mix.

2 Roll out puff pastry and using a 4 inch or 10cm round bowl cut the pastry into circles. Place mixture in the middle of the circle, then place another circle of pastry over the top. Using a fork press down the edges. Brush with egg yolk and then let it rest for 20 minutes. Then bake for 30-40 minutes in a moderate heat 180°C, 350°F, Gas Mark 4 until well risen and golden brown.

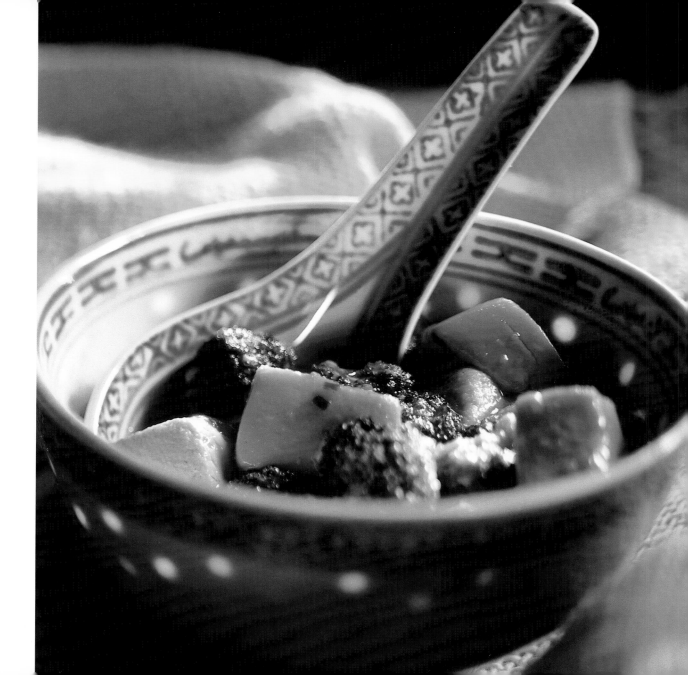

Preparation time 12 minutes
Marinating time 2-3 hours
Cooking time 4 minutes

Nutritional Content:
Energy 467 Kcal, 1950 kJ
Protein 32.70 g
Fat 30.06 g
Sodium 1.82 mmol
Potassium 16.20 mmol
Phosphorus 12.97 mmol

Barbequed Tofu

— SERVES 4 —
— PORTION SIZE 4oz/110g —

Tofu is made from beancurd, it can be bought in solid and soft varieties,
for this recipe I would recommend the solid type as it is easier to handle and cook.
The marinade will keep for weeks in the refrigerator.

INGREDIENTS

Tofu	1 lb/450g sliced or cubed
Toasted Ground Sesame Seeds	1 tbsp
Spring Onions	3 chopped
Garlic	4 cloves crushed
Sesame Oil	2 tbsp/30ml
Rice Wine or Sake	2 tbsp/30ml
Maple Syrup or Honey	2 tbsp/30ml
Black Pepper	pinch/2g
Soy Sauce	4 tbsp/60ml
Broccoli Florets	10

1 Stir or blend the onion, garlic, maple syrup, pepper, soy sauce, rice wine (or sake) and sesame seeds until thoroughly mixed.

2 Marinate the tofu in the sauce for several hours.

3 Fry or grill the tofu and serve with sauce and broccoli florets.

4 Serve with rice.

Preparation time 10 minutes
Cooking time 6-8 minutes

Nutritional Content:
Energy 292 Kcal, 1218 kJ
Protein 30.00 g
Fat 19.00 g
Sodium 6.00 mmol
Potassium 12.00 mmol
Phosphorus 10.00 mmol

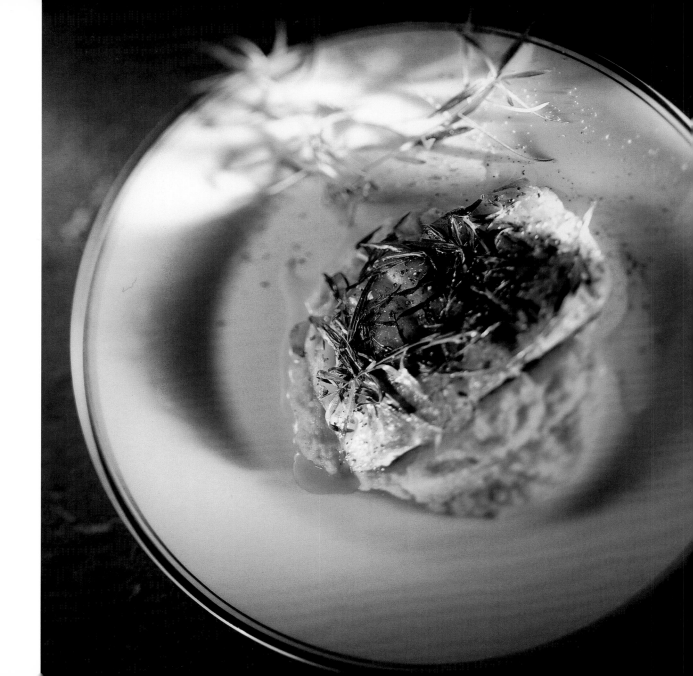

Peppered Tarragon Halibut with Anise Carrot Puree

Serve this with the Anise Carrot Puree on page 36.

INGREDIENTS

Olive Oil	4 tbsp/60ml
Halibut (fillet)	6 oz/170g x 4
Fresh Black Pepper	large pinch/4g
Fresh Tarragon	large pinch/4g

1 Heat olive oil in frying pan.

2 Season halibut with fresh cracked black pepper.

3 Pan fry on both sides in oil until cooked.

4 Finish with freshly chopped tarragon sprinkled over the halibut and serve.

Anise Carrot Puree

Preparation time 5 minutes
Cooking time 20 minutes

Nutritional Content:
Energy 154 Kcal, 633 kJ
Protein 0.86 g
Fat 15.29 g
Sodium 9.12 mmol
Potassium 3.57 mmol
Phosphorus 0.71 mmol

— SERVES 4 —

EQUIPMENT

Blender or potato masher.

INGREDIENTS

Medium Size Carrots	8 oz/225g
Olive Oil	2 floz/60ml
Shallots	2 chopped
Garlic	2 cloves chopped
Star Anise Powder	1 level tsp
	approximately
Salt	pinch/2g
Pepper	pinch/2g

1 Dice the carrots into small pieces.

2 Sweat the shallots and garlic in olive oil until soft and light brown, add the carrots and add enough water to barely cover, season lightly and bring to the boil. Cover with a lid and cook the carrots until soft and tender or until most of the liquid has evaporated.

3 Puree with a blender or use a potato masher, alternatively you can leave it chunky.

4 Add star anise powder a little at a time and keep tasting carrots, until correct flavour is obtained. Be careful not to over flavour the carrots with the star anise powder.

5 Serve as an accompaniment to Peppered Tarragon Halibut on page 34.

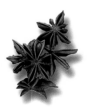

Five Spice Glazed Pork Chops

— SERVES 1 —

Five spice is a blend of spices that is used in Chinese cooking.

It is usually made from cinnamon, fennel, ginger, clove and pepper.

For variation other meats can be used but this will of course alter the nutritional analysis.

Preparation time 5 minutes
Cooking time 12-15 minutes
Marinating time 24 hours

Nutritional Content:
Energy 322 Kcal, 1350 kJ
Protein 39.70 g
Fat 16.24 g
Sodium 4.73 mmol
Potassium 18.58 mmol
Phosphorus 12.79 mmol

INGREDIENTS

Pork Chops	6 oz/170g
Chinese Five Spice	1 tsp
Brown Sugar	2 tsp
Pepper	pinch/2g
Olive Oil	2 tsp/10ml

1 Rub the Chinese Five Spice into the pork chops and leave to marinate for 24 hours.

2 To cook, preheat grill and place pork onto lightly oiled tray. The pork chops will take approximately 6-7 minutes each side depending on their thickness.

3 When nearly cooked sprinkle with brown sugar and caramelise under the grill until sugar bubbles and goes a deep brown colour.

Preparation time 24 hours including
marinating time
Cooking time 25 minutes

Nutritional Content:
Energy 1349 Kcal, 5599 kJ
Protein 74.36 g
Fat 101.87 g
Sodium 10.03 mmol
Potassium 32.69 mmol
Phosphorus 25.34 mmol

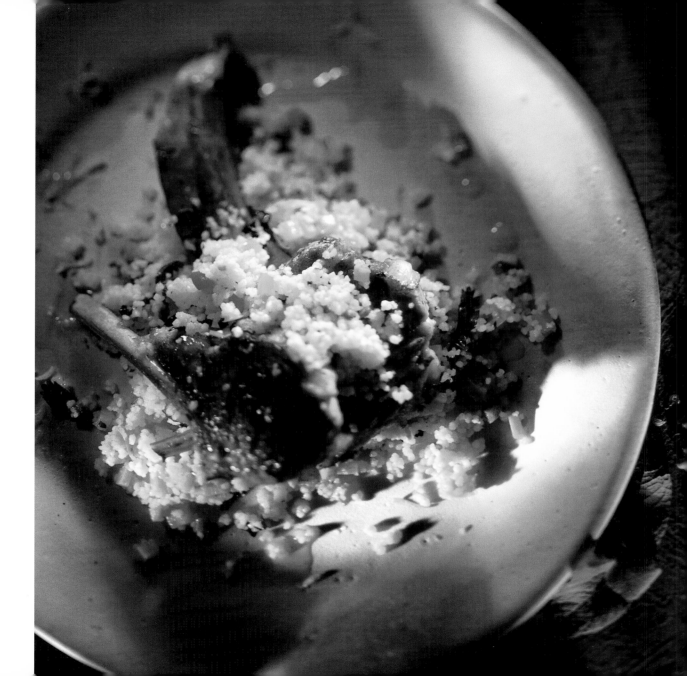

Grilled Lamb with Couscous Salad

*This is an easily prepared meal and makes something a little
special out of an ordinary cut of meat.*

INGREDIENTS

Lamb Cutlets	4 x 5 oz/140g
(or Lamb Neck Fillets or	
Lamb Chops)	
Fresh Mint	$^1/_2$ bunch chopped
Olive Oil	1 tbsp/15ml
Lemons	2
Instant Couscous	8 oz/225g
Red Pepper	1 diced
Green Pepper	1 diced
Yellow Pepper	1 diced
Carrots	2 diced
Coriander Seeds	$^1/_4$ tsp crushed
Cumin	$^1/_4$ tsp
Fresh Pepper	pinch/2g
Garlic	3 cloves chopped
Fresh Coriander	2 tbsp chopped

1 Marinate lamb in chopped garlic, mint, olive oil and juice
of 1 lemon for at least 3-4 hours or 24 hours if possible.

2 To prepare instant couscous cover with boiling water for
a few minutes, until it puffs up, or follow instructions on
the packet.

3 Gently fry the mixed peppers and carrots in olive oil.
Add the crushed coriander seeds, cumin and the juice of
remaining lemon. Gently combine this mixture with the
couscous.

4 Grill chops under a hot grill until cooked to your liking.

5 Add the chopped coriander to the couscous and serve
with the grilled lamb on top.

Preparation time 15 minutes
Cooking time 10 minutes

Nutritional Content:
Energy 103 Kcal, 425 kJ
Protein 1.20 g
Fat 6.70 g
Sodium 5.03 mmol
Potassium 0.94 mmol
Phosphorus 0.05 mmol

VARIATIONS

The analysis is based on the cream cheese being added. If you omit this, it will change the analysis as will adding different herbs and vegetables.

EQUIPMENT

Loaf tin.
Cling film.

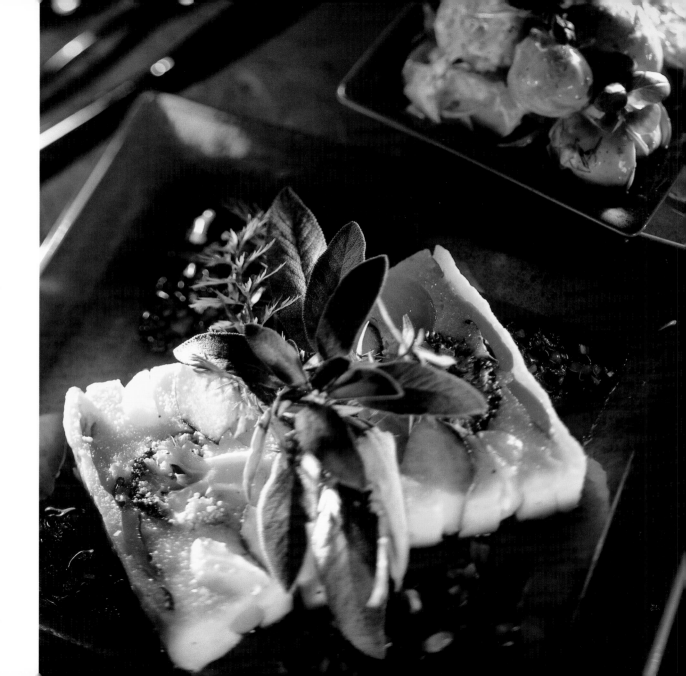

Polenta Terrine

*Polenta can be made and stored in the fridge and then served in salads or with meat and fish.
As well as the cheese which has been suggested as a flavouring, why not experiment with your favourite herbs or layer
it with lightly cooked vegetables (remember this will change the nutritional analysis). For an easy accompaniment to a
summer barbecue it can also be brushed with oil and then barbecued or skewered and used as a kebab ingredient.*

INGREDIENTS

Butter	6 oz/170g
Water	2¹/₂ pint/1.5 litres
Polenta (instant Cornmeal)	13 oz/370g
Extra Virgin Olive Oil	3 tbsp/45ml
White Peppercorn	pinch/2g
	freshly milled
Salt	1 tsp
Grated Nutmeg	pinch/2g
Cream Cheese - optional	1 oz/28g

1 **Preparing Polenta:** Bring water to the boil with nutmeg, butter and salt if required.

2 Pour in polenta and mix thoroughly for about 5-10 minutes.

3 If using cream cheese or other seasoning it can be mixed in at the last minute.

4 Pour polenta into lightly oiled tray and cool. When cold take out and slice into squares or rectangles and grill or lightly flour and pan fry in olive oil and butter.

1 **Making a terrine:** Cooked broccoli, button onions, courgettes and carrots (both cut lengthways), green beans and baby sweetcorn. All these vegetables are suitable for a terrine or any other low potassium vegetable (see page 77), but remember to add the analysis of the vegetables to the dish.

2 All vegetables must be cooked beforehand in boiling water then refreshed under ice cold water to prevent from further cooking, then dried.

3 Lightly oil a terrine or loaf tin then line with cling film, this makes the turning out of the terrine more easy.

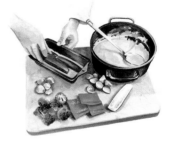

Making a terrine

4 To assemble the terrine have the polenta warm and pour a thin layer into the bottom of the tin. Then arrange a layer of vegetables, cover this layer with more polenta and repeat until the terrine is full. Cover with cling film and chill for several hours until firm to the touch or it can be made the day before you need it. Once turned out slice and serve.

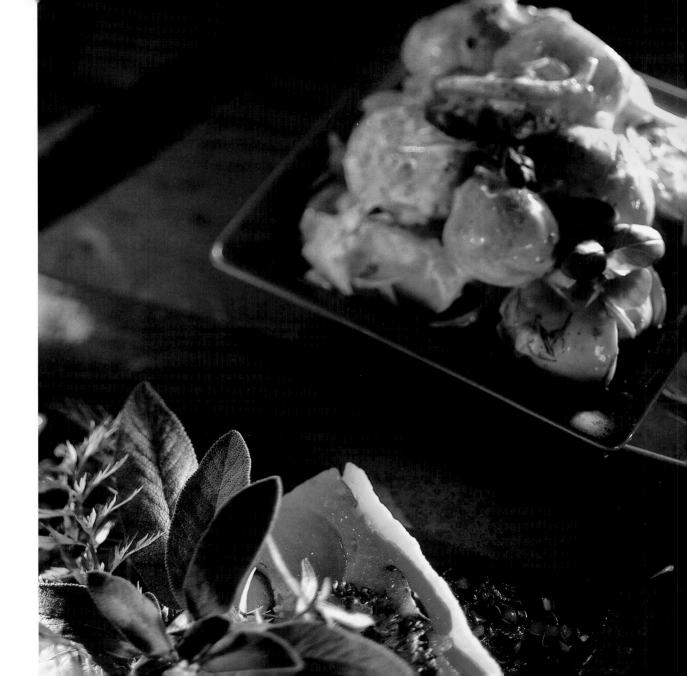

Preparation time 10 minutes
Cooking time 15 minutes

Nutritional Content:
Energy 328 Kcal, 1369 kJ
Protein 3.25 g
Fat 21.00 g
Sodium 6.00 mmol
Potassium 12.00 mmol
Phosphorus 2.00 mmol

Red Onion, Basil and Potato Salad

— SERVES 4 —
— PORTION SIZE 3½ oz/100g —

This is a good accompaniment to barbecued food and the added basil makes a nice change from the traditional potato salad.

INGREDIENTS

Baby Potatoes	1½ lb/680g
Red Onion	4 oz/110g
Basil	12 leaves
Pepper	large pinch/4g
Mayonnaise	4 oz/110g

1 Place your potatoes into a pan filled with cold water and bring to the boil.

2 Boil potatoes for approximately 15 minutes, check they are cooked by prodding them with the end of a sharp knife. The knife should easily penetrate the flesh when they are cooked. Cool in cold water and strain.

3 Cut potatoes in half.

4 Finely chop the onion and basil.

5 Add all ingredients to the potatoes and mix together well and serve.

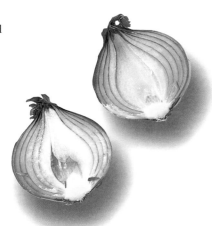

Tarragon and Mustard Butter

Preparation time 5 minutes

Nutritional Content:
Energy 213 Kcal, 876 kJ
Protein 0.48 g
Fat 23.36 g
Sodium 11.82 mmol
Potassium 0.46 mmol
Phosphorus 0.48 mmol

- SERVES 8 -
- PORTION SIZE 1 oz / 28g -

Serve with grilled white meat or fish.

STORAGE

Refrigerate or freeze.

EQUIPMENT

Greaseproof paper.

INGREDIENTS

Unsalted Butter	8 oz / 225g
Tarragon	1 bunch chopped
Grain Mustard	4 heaped tsp
Fresh White Pepper	pinch / 2g
Lemon	1

1 Soften butter.

2 Add chopped tarragon, mustard and the juice of the lemon, season with pepper.

3 Open a large square of greaseproof paper. Place the butter in the centre in a sausage shape and roll in greaseproof tightly. Refrigerate or freeze and use as required.

Hollandaise Sauce

— SERVES 6 —

*A basic sauce recipe that will dress any simple grilled fish for dinner.
To make Béarnaise sauce that is excellent with grilled meats just add chopped
tarragon, chervil and parsley to the basic Hollandaise sauce.*

Preparation time 15 minutes
Cooking time 10 minutes

Nutritional Content:
Energy 316 Kcal, 1300 kJ
Protein 2.12 g
Fat 33.80 g
Sodium 12.72 mmol
Potassium 1.78 mmol
Phosphorus 2.38 mmol

INGREDIENTS

Egg Yolks	3
Unsalted Butter	8 oz/225g
Whole White Peppercorns	8-10
Thyme	1 sprig
Bay Leaf	1
White Wine Vinegar	1/4 pint/150ml
Cayenne	pinch/2g
Lemon	1/2 juice of
Shallots	2 chopped

1 Melt butter on stove slowly, or put into the microwave and melt.

2 Finely chop shallots, place into saucepan with crushed peppercorns. Add thyme, bay leaf and white wine vinegar and bring to boil. Reduce down until nearly all the vinegar has evaporated.

3 Take off the heat and allow to cool for a few minutes. Add the egg yolks and whisk over gentle heat (ideally a saucepan of boiling water: the steam being sufficient heat).

4 The egg yolks will start to become frothy, light and thicken. Take off the heat and allow to cool.

5 Test the temperature of the butter, it should be luke warm. Whisk gently into the eggs in a steady stream. If the mixture starts to thicken too much, add some warm water to thin it down slightly.

6 Add all the butter then season with lemon juice and pinch of cayenne.

7 The shallots and peppercorns can be left in the sauce, but if you want you can pass the Hollandaise through a sieve or squeeze through a piece of muslin.

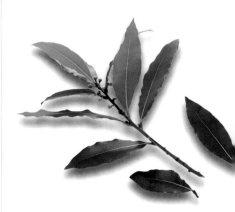

45

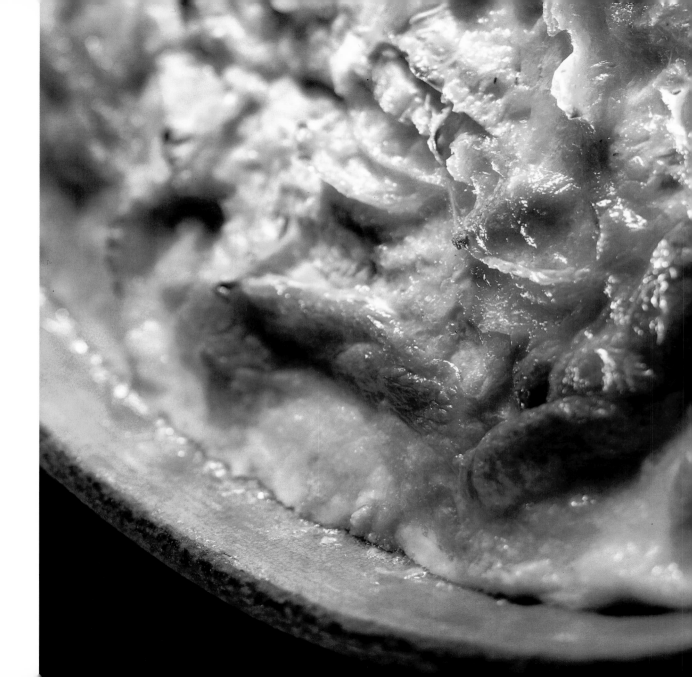

Preparation time 20 minutes
Cooking time 30-40 minutes

Nutritional Content:
Energy 74 Kcal, 304 kJ
Protein 0.65 g
Fat 7.26 g
Sodium 2.45 mmol
Potassium 3.42 mmol
Phosphorus 0.80 mmol

— ■ —

EQUIPMENT

Earthenware dish.

— ■ —

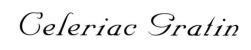

Celeriac Gratin

— SERVES 6 —
— PORTION SIZE 7 oz / 200g —

INGREDIENTS

Butter	2 oz/55g
Celeriac	2 lb/900g
	finely sliced
Onion	7 oz/200g
	finely sliced
Double Cream	15 floz/450ml
Garlic	1 oz/28g
Salt	pinch/2g
Pepper	large pinch/4g

1 Grease and season an earthenware dish, cook onion slices in a saucepan without fat until transparent.

2 Bring the cream and half of the garlic to the boil then simmer for approximately 10-15 minutes. Chop the rest of the garlic.

3 Lay the celeriac in layers in the dish with the chopped garlic and cooked onions in between each layer. Approximately 6-8 layers in total.

4 Pour infused cream over the top of the layers until just covering top layer. Bake in oven for approximately 35-45 minutes at a moderate heat of 180-200°C, 350-400°F, Gas Mark 4-6.

Preparation time 10 minutes
Cooking time 30 minutes

Nutritional Content:
Energy 491 Kcal, 2023 kJ
Protein 4.13 g
Fat 49.19 g
Sodium 16.38 mmol
Potassium 11.19 mmol
Phosphorus 0.37 mmol

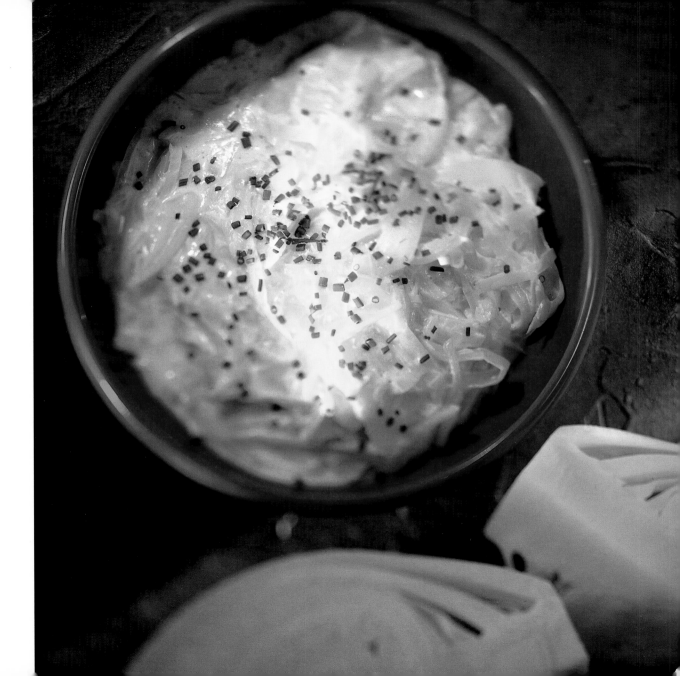

White Cabbage with Cream Cheese

INGREDIENTS

White Cabbage	8 oz/225g thinly sliced
Onion	1/60g sliced
Butter	2 oz/55g
Cream Cheese	4 oz/110g
White Pepper	pinch/2g

1 Place cabbage and onion in saucepan with butter and cook gently with tight fitting lid, being careful not to colour the cabbage. Stirring occasionally will help to prevent this.

2 When cabbage is soft and tender, approximately 20-25 minutes cooking time, take off the heat and add cream cheese. Season with fresh white pepper and serve.

Preparation time 25-30 minutes
Cooking time 10 minutes

Nutritional Content:
Energy 378 Kcal, 1576 kJ
Protein 12 g
Fat 23.70 g
Sodium 26.50 mmol
Potassium 10.70 mmol
Phosphorus 7.00 mmol

VARIATIONS

If you have been advised to follow
a low potassium diet and if this
dish is served as a starter it
should be followed by a low
potassium main course.

EQUIPMENT

Food processor or liquidiser.

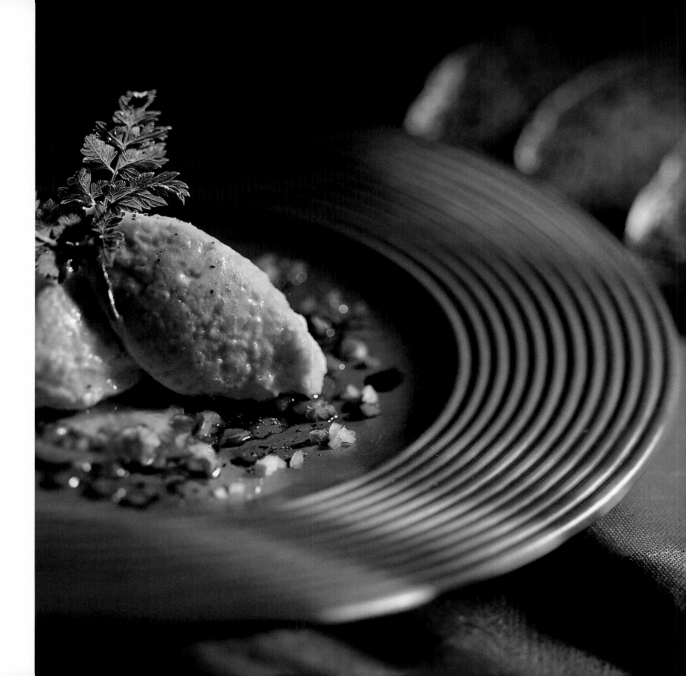

Spiced Cod Mousse with Red Onion and Tomato Salad

— SERVES 6 —

— PORTION SIZE ½ oz/15g —

This recipe has its roots in the salt cod dish that is served in Portugal,

needless to say the original version is not acceptable due to the high salt content.

This makes a piquant alternative and can be served as a starter or light snack.

INGREDIENTS

Cod	6 oz/170g boned and skinned
Garlic	2 cloves
Cooked White Rice	7 oz/200g
Egg Yolk	1
Single Cream	12 floz/350ml
Worcestershire Sauce	splash
Tabasco	splash
Olive Oil	4 tbsp/60ml
Lemon	1
Freshly Milled Black Pepper	pinch/2g
Tomato	3 sliced
Red Onions	1 chopped
Balsamic Vinegar	4 tbsp/60ml
Salt	1 tsp
Ground White Pepper	1 tsp
Wholemeal Toast	6 slices

1 Crush garlic, add to cod and then place in pan, add sufficient water to cover and then poach for 10 minutes. Remove from water and leave to cool.

2 Using a food processor or liquidiser mix rice, egg yolk and cream and half of the cod, to a smooth mixture. Season with Worcestershire sauce, a splash of tabasco and salt.

3 Add a little lemon juice and fresh pepper and blend again with a little olive oil (3 tbsps).

4 In a separate bowl break up the remaining cod into flakes and then gently add the blended fish mixture. Cover and refrigerate.

5 Bring a pan of water to the boil.

6 De-core the tomatoes and dip into the boiling water for approximately 10 seconds. Remove and plunge into ice water. Peel off skin, slice tomatoes and arrange on a plate in a circle. Sprinkle with the finely chopped red onion, balsamic vinegar, a little olive oil (1 tbsp between the 6 servings), and a twist of fresh black pepper.

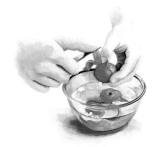

Peeling a tomato.

7 Dip two dessert spoons into boiling hot water then spoon out some cod mixture and shape into quenelles using the two spoons. Place on top of tomato and onion and serve with wholemeal toast.

Preparation time 5 minutes
Cooking time 12-15 minutes

Nutritional Content:
Energy 500 Kcal, 2085 kJ
Protein 65.80 g
Fat 25.90 g
Sodium 6.30 mmol
Potassium 26.00 mmol
Phosphorus 20.00 mmol

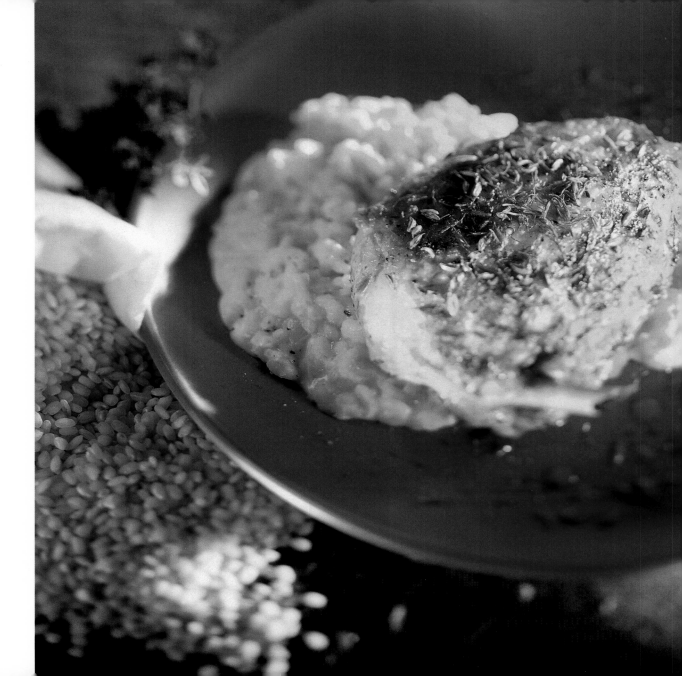

Saffron and Rosemary Crusted Chicken

This recipe uses only a few ingredients to make a simple but impressive main course.
The chicken can be covered in the seasoning in advance and kept refrigerated
until it needs to be cooked. This will save time at the last minute.

INGREDIENTS

Chicken Breast with skin	1 x 8 oz/225g
Saffron	large pinch/4g
Fresh Rosemary	1 tsp
Freshly Milled Black Pepper	pinch/2g
Olive Oil	2 tsp/10mls

1 Sprinkle chicken breast with saffron and rosemary.

2 Gently pan fry in olive oil until cooked. The meat is cooked when it is firm to the touch and the juices run clear.

3 To serve, you can sprinkle some more saffron onto the chicken breast.

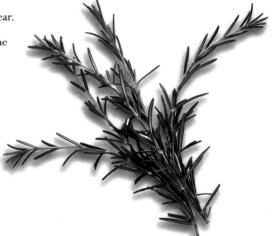

Preparation time 20 minutes
Cooking time 45 minutes

Nutritional Content:
Energy 573 Kcal, 2393 kJ
Protein 6.64 g
Fat 35.61 g
Sodium 41.26 mmol
Potassium 6.10 mmol
Phosphorus 4.05 mmol

Saffron Risotto

— SERVES 4 —

— PORTION SIZE 7 oz / 200 g —

Risottos have made a come back in recent years. They are easy to prepare and cook and can be made from ingredients that are often already in the cupboard. This risotto is no exception. For a slightly different taste and texture it can also be made with Basmati rice.

INGREDIENTS

Onion	1 finely chopped
Garlic	2 cloves crushed
Thyme	large pinch/4g
Saffron	large pinch/4g
Fresh Chicken/Vegetable Stock or use ½ a stock cube	1 pint/600ml
Arborio Rice	9 oz/255g
Fresh Milled White Pepper	pinch/2g
Bay Leaf	1
Salt	pinch/2g
Cream Cheese	4 oz/110g
Double Cream	5 floz/150ml

1 Sweat onions in olive oil with garlic, thyme and saffron.

2 Moisten with some of the stock. Add rice and cook gently for a few minutes.

3 Add the rest of the stock, pepper and bay leaf.

4 Cook gently and slowly, stirring occasionally so rice does not stick.

5 Rice should be quite wet in consistency (sauce like). Add more stock if needed.

6 Finish with cream cheese plus a little double cream if you desire.

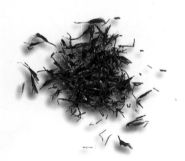

Crispy Grilled Lemon Sole with Garlic Lemon Oil, Ginger and Mint

— SERVES 4 —

This dish can be served as a main course of one fillet per person and served with plain buttered pasta

Preparation time 25 minutes
Cooking time 10-15 minutes

Nutritional Content:
Energy 683 Kcal, 2835 kJ
Protein 26.17 g
Fat 54.89 g
Sodium 8.00 mmol
Potassium 10.00 mmol
Phosphorus 10.00 mmol

INGREDIENTS

Lemon Sole	4 x 5 oz/140g fillets skinned
Flour	2 oz/55g
Unsalted Butter (melted)	4 oz/110g
Breadcrumbs	2 oz/55g
Lemon Juice and Zest	1
Garlic	1 clove finely chopped
Olive Oil	3¹/₂ floz/100ml
Mint	2 tsp chopped
Ginger	1 tsp cut into thin strips
Coriander Seeds	¹/₂ tsp
Fresh Pepper	pinch/2g

1 Lightly score with a sharp knife the fillets of sole on the skin side. This will stop the fillets from curling up when cooking.

2 Season the fish with pepper and dip into the flour, then dip into the previously melted butter before finally coating with breadcrumbs, which have been mixed with grated lemon and chopped mint. Place the fillets onto a lightly greased tray.

3 Sweat the ginger, garlic and crushed coriander seeds in the olive oil being careful not to colour. Then pour in lemon juice and take off the heat. Set aside and keep warm.

4 Grill the fillets under a pre-heated grill for approximately 8-10 minutes on one side only until golden brown. Serve on warm plates with the dressing around and garnish with freshly picked mint.

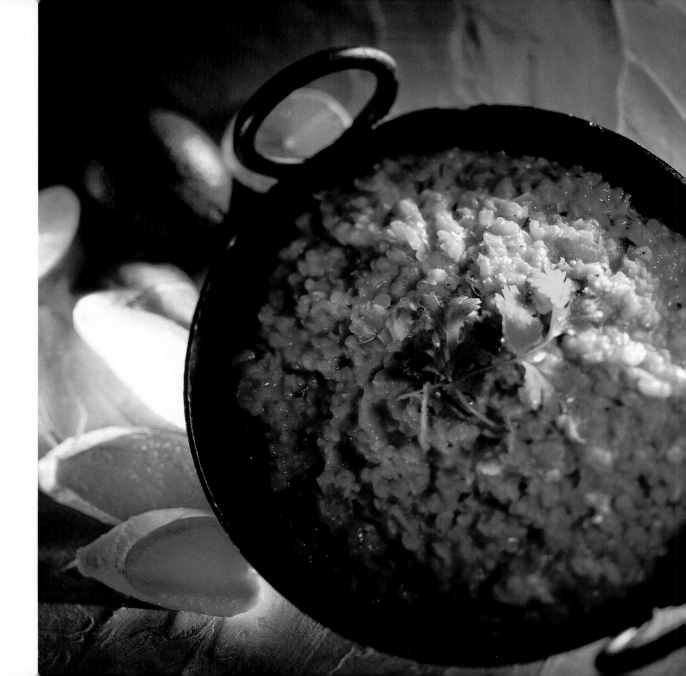

Preparation time 15 minutes
Cooking time 35-40 minutes

Nutritional Content:
Energy 379 Kcal, 1590 kJ
Protein 16.16 g
Fat 17.67 g
Sodium 12.48 mmol
Potassium 22.00 mmol
Phosphorus 8.60 mmol

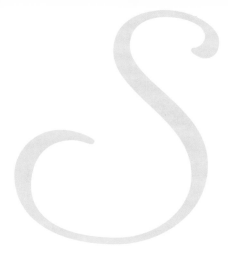

Spiced Red Lentils

— SERVES 4 —
— PORTION SIZE 3½ oz / 100g —

INGREDIENTS

Red Lentils	8 oz/225g
Onion	2 chopped
Butter	3 oz/85g
Garlic	6 cloves sliced
Carrot	1 medium grated
Cumin Seeds	2 tsp
Yellow Mustard Seeds	1½ tsp
Turmeric	2 tsp
Coconut Milk	8 floz/250ml
Fresh Ginger	4-5 thick slices unpeeled
Lime Juice and Zest	1
Water	10 floz/300ml
Sugar	1 tsp
Salt	pinch/2g
Fresh Milled Black Pepper	pinch/2g

1 Sweat onions until slightly brown, add the garlic, carrot and cumin seeds. Allow to cook gently for 3 minutes.

2 Stir in the turmeric and lentils and add the water, coconut milk and ginger.

3 Cook gently for 25-30 minutes or until lentils are tender.

4 Add the lime juice and zest, season with salt and pepper. At the last minutes add the freshly chopped coriander.

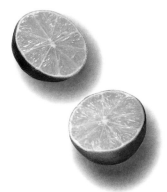

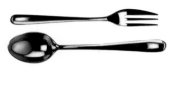

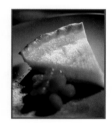

Desserts

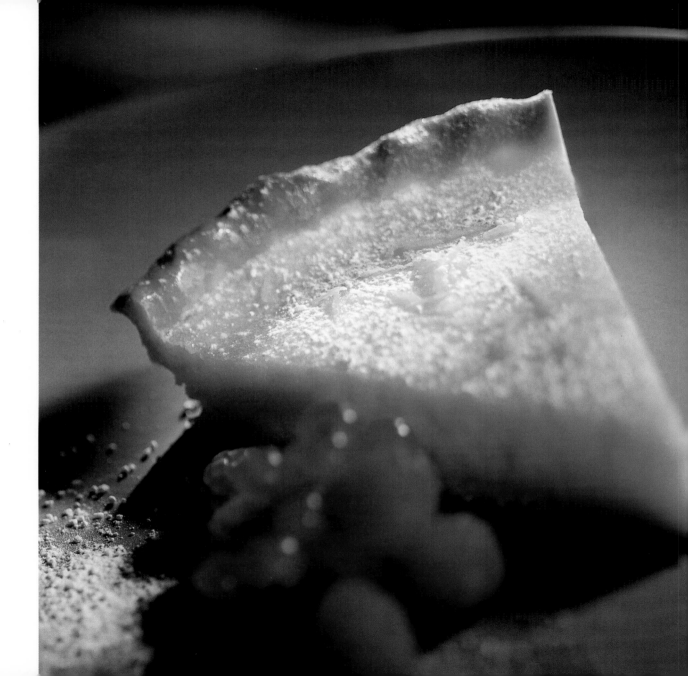

Preparation time 35 minutes
Cooking time 50 minutes

Nutritional Content:
Energy 107 Kcal, 449 kJ
Protein 2.00 g
Fat 6.50 g
Sodium 2.00 mmol
Potassium 0.75 mmol
Phosphorus 0.87 mmol

EQUIPMENT

10 inch or 25cm flan ring.

Greaseproof paper.

Baking beans or rice.

Lemon Tart

This is a rich dessert and so it can follow a plain
main course to make a luscious end to a meal.

INGREDIENTS

For the Pastry

Eggs	2
Caster Sugar	4 oz/110g
Butter	10 oz/285g
Soft Plain Flour	1¼ lb/570g
Salt (optional)	pinch/2g

For the Filling

Eggs	6
Double Cream	8 floz/250ml
Caster Sugar	5 oz/140g
Lemons	2

1 **For the Pastry:** Cream the eggs and sugar together until smooth. Add the butter and mix for a few minutes. Take care not to over soften the butter.

2 Gradually incorporate the sieved flour and salt, mixing until smooth. Allow to rest in fridge for at least 1 hour before using.

3 Grease a 10 inch (25cm) flan ring and place onto a baking sheet. Roll out pastry and line the flan ring and trim the edges. Bake blind (cover the pastry with greaseproof paper and fill with rice or beans) for 5-8 minutes at a moderate heat of 180-200°C, 350-400°F, Gas Mark 4-6.

4 Take out the greaseproof paper and brush the pastry with a little beaten egg yolk, put flan ring back into the oven for a further 2-3 minutes to give it a glaze. This acts as a sealant to the pastry so when the lemon cream is poured into the pastry case it does not leak or go soggy.

1 **For the Filling:** Beat the eggs and sugar together.

2 Warm the cream in a pan and gently bring it nearly to the boil.

3 Add the cream to the egg mixture.

4 Add the lemon juice and mix well.

5 Pour the lemon filling into the flan ring and bake for approximately 35-45 minutes on a low oven of 140°C, 250°F, Gas Mark 1.

Preparation time 5 minutes
Cooking time 10 -15 minutes

Nutritional Content:
Energy 357 Kcal, 1503 kJ
Protein 3.54 g
Fat 13.22 g
Sodium 8.29 mmol
Potassium 1.63 mmol
Phosphorus 1.16 mmol

EQUIPMENT

Baking Tray.

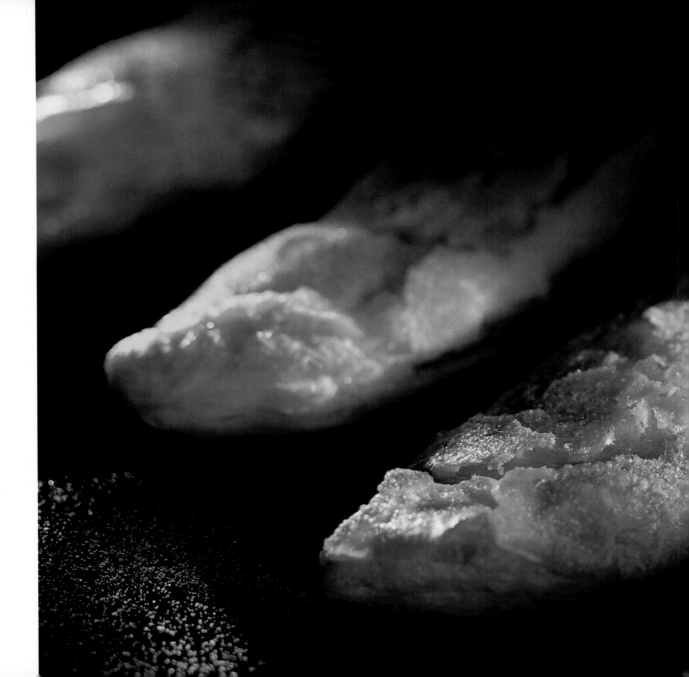

Jam Turnovers

— SERVES 4 —
— PORTION SIZE 7 oz/200g —

*These Turnovers are quick and easy to make with ingredients
that you can keep in the freezer and cupboard. Just right for a teatime treat.*

INGREDIENTS

Puff Pastry	8 oz/225g
Jam	8 oz/225g
Double Cream Whipped	4 tbsp/60ml

1 Roll out the pastry to a thickness of 0.5cm ($\frac{1}{4}$ inch).

2 Cut with a fancy cutter into 10cm diameter (4 inch) rounds. A saucer or small side plate will do if you don't have the right sized cutter.

3 Roll out until slightly oval 12x10cm (5x4 inches). Moisten the edges.

4 Place a little jam in the centre of each. Fold over and seal firmly.

5 Brush with egg white and sprinkle with caster sugar.

6 Place sugar side up on a greased baking sheet. Bake in a hot oven (220ºC, 425ºF, Gas Mark 7) for approximately 15-20 minutes.

7 Serve with double cream.

Lemon Meringue Pie

Preparation time 25 minutes
Cooking time 25 minutes

Nutritional Content:
Energy 496 Kcal, 2086 kJ
Protein 5.74 g
Fat 20.31 g
Sodium 11.29 mmol
Potassium 2.34 mmol
Phosphorus 2.54 mmol

— SERVES 8 —

EQUIPMENT

8 inch or 20cm flan ring.

Greaseproof paper.

Baking beans or rice.

INGREDIENTS

For the Pastry

Eggs	2
Caster Sugar	2 oz/55g
Butter	5 oz/140g
Soft Plain Flour	8 oz/225g
Salt (optional)	pinch/2g

For the Filling

Egg Yolks	2
Egg Whites	4
Caster Sugar	12 oz/340g
Lemon	1
Butter	1 oz/28g
Cornflour	1 oz/28g
Water	1/4 pint/150ml

1 **For the Pastry:** Cream the eggs and sugar together until smooth. Add the butter and mix for a few minutes.

2 Gradually incorporate the sieved flour and salt, mixing until smooth. Allow to rest in fridge for at least 1 hour before using.

3 Grease a flan ring and place onto a baking sheet. Roll out pastry and line an 8 inch (20cm) flan ring and trim the edges. Bake blind (cover the pastry with greaseproof paper and fill with rice or beans) for 5-8 minutes at a moderate heat of 180-200°C, 350-400°F, Gas Mark 4-6.

4 Take out the greaseproof paper and brush the pastry with a little beaten egg yolk, put flan ring back into the oven for a further 2-3 minutes to give it a glaze. This acts as a sealant.

5 **For the Filling:** Prepare the lemon curd by boiling the water, sugar, zest and juice of the lemon to a syrup. Thicken with diluted cornflour, remove from the heat, add the butter and whisk in yolks. Place in the flan case.

6 Whisk the egg whites until stiff then fold in the 8oz caster sugar. Pipe or spread on the lemon filling and bake in the oven 220°C, 425°F, Gas Mark 7 for 10-15 minutes.

Lemon Cream Cheese Pound Cake

— SERVES 6 —

Preparation time 20 minutes
Cooking time 1¼ - 1½ hours

Nutritional Content:
Energy 916 Kcal, 3853 kJ
Protein 9.33 g
Fat 40.93 g
Sodium 23.66 mmol
Potassium 4.24 mmol
Phosphorus 9.47 mmol

EQUIPMENT

A deep 9 inch or 23cm cake tin.

Wire cooling rack.

INGREDIENTS

White Sugar	1½ lb/680g
Butter	8 oz/225g
Cream Cheese	8 oz/225g softened
Lemon Juice	1 tbsp/15ml
Vanilla Extract	1 tbsp/15ml
Lemon Extract	1 tsp/5ml
Orange Extract	½ tsp/2.5ml
Nutmeg	¼ tsp
Salt	⅛ tsp
Eggs	6
Plain Flour	12 oz/340g

For the Lemon Icing

Icing Sugar	4 oz/110g
Sugar	2 tbsp
Lemon Extract	¼ tsp/1ml

Yellow food colouring if desired

1 Grease and flour a deep 9 inch (23cm) cake tin.

2 In a large bowl beat the white sugar, butter and cream cheese until light and fluffy.

3 Beat in lemon juice, vanilla extract, lemon extract, orange extract, nutmeg and salt.

4 Add eggs, one at a time, beating well after each addition. Add flour and beat until smooth.

5 Pour batter into prepared cake tin. Bake at 160°C, 325°F, Gas Mark 3 for 1¼ - 1½ hours until golden brown and when a skewer inserted into the centre comes out clean. Cool in the tin for 10 minutes.

6 With a metal spatula, loosen the cake from the tin and invert onto wire rack to cool completely.

7 **For the Icing:** Prepare icing by combining the sugars and enough water to make a smooth glaze.

8 Add lemon extract and the food colouring. Spread icing over the cake, allowing some to drizzle down the sides.

Preparation time 25 minutes
Cooking time 45 - 50 minutes

Nutritional Content:
Energy 297 Kcal, 1242 kJ
Protein 3.46 g
Fat 16.51 g
Sodium 9.86 mmol
Potassium 5.87 mmol
Phosphorus 1.80 mmol

EQUIPMENT

8 inch or 20cm size cake tin.

Wire cooling rack.

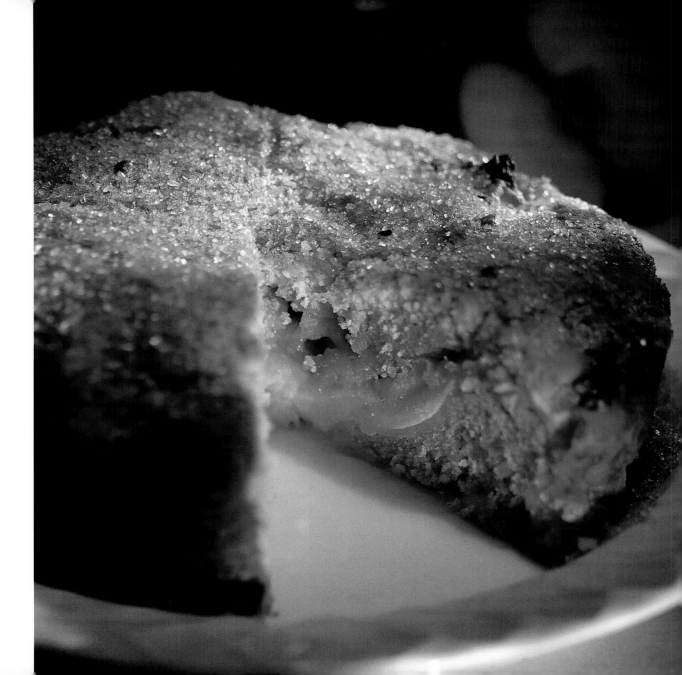

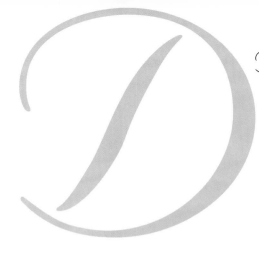

Devonshire Apple Cake

— SERVES 8 —

This cake is delicious served on its own or with a small helping of ice cream, custard or crème fraîche.

INGREDIENTS

Plain Flour	6 oz/170g
Caster Sugar	4 oz/110g
Cream of Tartar	1½ tsp
Bicarbonate of Soda	1½ tsp
Unsalted Butter	4 oz/110g
Cooking Apples	4 cored and finely chopped
Egg	1
Skimmed Milk	5 floz/150ml
Ground Cinnamon	1½ tsp
Brown Sugar	1 tsp

1 Line the bottom of an 8 inch or 20cm cake tin with waxed paper. Butter and flour. Preheat oven to 180°C, 350°F, Gas Mark 4.

2 Sift flour, sugar and baking powder into a large bowl. With a pastry blender or knife, cut in butter until mixture resembles fine breadcrumbs.

3 Toss chopped apple in cinnamon and then add to flour mixture. Set aside.

4 In small bowl, whisk together egg and milk until blended. Stir into apple mixture until mixed (batter will be stiff). Spread batter evenly in the tin.

5 Bake in preheated oven for 45-50 minutes. Sprinkle brown sugar over the top approximately 5 minutes before the end of cooking time. Continue cooking until a skewer, when inserted in the centre comes out clean.

6 Remove from oven. Cool for 10 minutes in the tin before removing and allowing to cool on a wire rack.

Nutritional Content:
Energy 378 Kcal, 1580 kJ
Protein 5.92 g
Fat 23.15 g
Sodium 5.45 mmol
Potassium 5.81 mmol
Phosphorus 4.43 mmol

EQUIPMENT

2 pint/1.2 litre pudding basin.

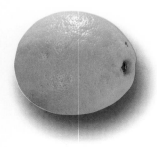

Steamed Lemon Sponge Pudding

‐ SERVES 6 ‐

A traditional pudding that is enjoyed by everyone.
The cooking time can be reduced by pressure cooking the sponge,
(see the manufacturer's instructions for your pressure cooker for cooking times).

INGREDIENTS

Unsalted Butter	4 oz/110g
Caster or Brown Sugar	4 oz/110g
Eggs	2
Flour, White or Wholemeal	6 oz/170g
Bicarbonate of Soda	1 tsp
Cream of Tartar	1 tsp
Skimmed Milk	2-3 floz/60-90ml
Lemons	2

1 Grease a pudding basin.

2 Cream the butter and sugar together until fluffy and almost white. Add a few drops of lemon juice to the creamed mixture.

3 Gradually add the beaten eggs, if mixture begins to curdle add a little flour.

4 Gently fold in sieved flour mixture, adding a little milk if needed in order to keep the mixture to a dropping consistency.

5 Place in pudding basin and cover securely with greased greaseproof paper. Place the basin in a large pan, fill the pan with cold water to half way up the basin, cover with a lid and bring to the boil. When boiling reduce the heat so the water keeps simmering and steam for 1-1¹/₂ hours. Keep checking on the level of the water and top up if water level is dropping. Before you turn out the pudding let it stand for 5-10 minutes.

Peach Crumble

— SERVES 4 —

Preparation time 10 minutes
Cooking time 25 - 30 minutes

Nutritional Content:
Energy 385 Kcal, 1616 kJ
Protein 5.27 g
Fat 17.87 g
Sodium 7.90 mmol
Potassium 6.96 mmol
Phosphorus 3.60 mmol

EQUIPMENT

Ovenproof dish.

INGREDIENTS

Tinned Peaches	14 oz/400g
(in natural juice)	drained
Wholemeal Flour	3 oz/85g
White Flour	3 oz/85g
Butter or Margarine	3 oz/85g
Sugar	2 oz/55g

1 Place peaches into a greased ovenproof dish

2 Sieve the flour into a mixing bowl. Add the chilled, diced butter or margarine and rub into the flour until a fine breadcrumb consistency is reached. Mix in the sugar.

3 Place the crumble mixture on top of the fruit.

4 Bake in a moderate oven 200°C, 400°F, Gas Mark 6 for 25-30 minutes.

Preparation time 5 minutes
Hob cooking time 15 minutes
Oven cooking time 2-2 $\frac{1}{2}$ hours

Nutritional Content:
Energy 289 Kcal, 1218 kJ
Protein 8.77 g
Fat 10.21 g
Sodium 5.46 mmol
Potassium 8.17 mmol
Phosphorus 7.62 mmol

VARIATIONS

For a change serve with
tinned fruit.

EQUIPMENT

Earthenware dish.

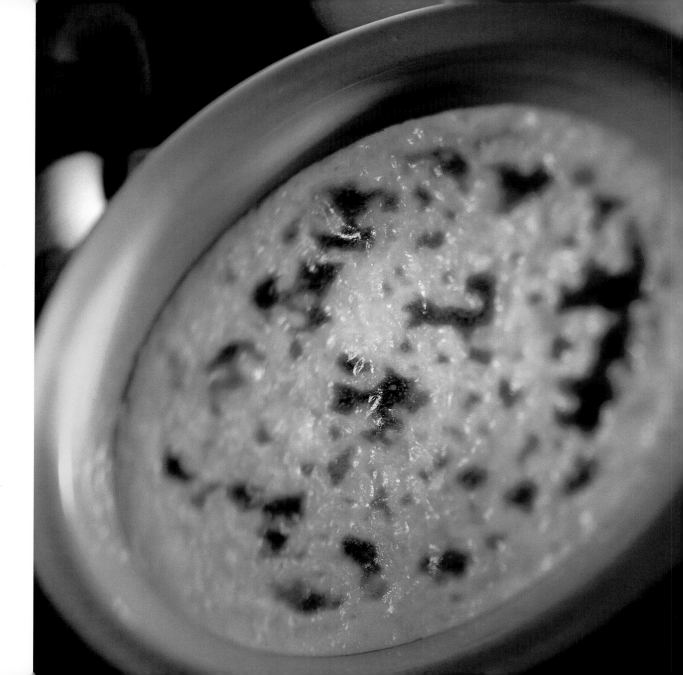

Glazed Rice Pudding

— SERVES 4 —
— PORTION SIZE 6 oz / 170g —

This is a simple rice pudding that is really good served just as it is.
It can be made on the hob or in the oven depending on the amount of cooking time that you have.
To make a change serve this with tinned fruit.

INGREDIENTS

Carolina Rice (pudding rice)	4 oz/110g
Caster Sugar	2 oz/55g
Milk (skimmed)	1 pint/600ml
Butter	1/2 oz/15g
Vanilla Essence	2-3 drops
Grated Nutmeg	pinch/2g
Ground Cinnamon	1/4 tsp
Egg Yolk	1
Half Fat Cream	1/4 pint/150ml

1 **Hob Method:** Put rice, milk and sugar into a large thick bottomed pan. Add the vanilla, nutmeg, cinnamon and butter.

2 Cook gently until rice is cooked and has absorbed the milk. Add more milk if necessary. To avoid the rice sticking stir regularly.

3 Gently beat the egg yolk and cream together. Add to rice pudding, take off the heat and add more sugar if desired.

4 Pour into a buttered earthenware dish and glaze under a hot grill until brown, then serve.

1 **Oven Method:** Grease ovenproof dish with half of the butter.

2 Put rice, milk, sugar, vanilla, nutmeg and cinnamon into the dish.

3 Dot with the remaining butter.

4 Cook in oven at 150°C, 300°F , Gas Mark 2 for 2-2 1/2 hours.

5 Gently beat egg yolk and cream together. Add to rice pudding, add more sugar if desired. Glaze under a hot grill until brown, then serve.

Preparation time 20 minutes
Cooking time 45 minutes

Nutritional Content:
Energy 390 Kcal, 1639 kJ
Protein 10.41 g
Fat 17.07 g
Sodium 14.31 mmol
Potassium 7.54 mmol
Phosphorus 6.43 mmol

EQUIPMENT

Earthenware dish.

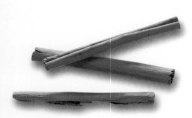

Pear and Grand Marnier Bread and Butter Pudding

— SERVES 6 —

INGREDIENTS

Sliced White Bread	8-9 slices
Tinned Pears	14 oz/400g
Skimmed Milk	1 pint/600ml
Ground Nutmeg	$\frac{1}{2}$ tsp
Ground Cinnamon	$\frac{1}{2}$ tsp
Vanilla (fresh if possible)	few drops
Eggs	3
Caster Sugar	2 oz/55g
Grand Marnier	2-3 tbsp/30-45mls
Unsalted Butter	$2\frac{1}{2}$ oz/70g

1 Lightly butter earthenware or ovenproof dish.

2 Butter bread then remove crusts and cut into triangles. Thinly slice tinned pears. Layer dish with bread, followed by a layer of pears, then bread.

3 Bring milk nearly to boil. Add nutmeg, cinnamon and vanilla.

4 Whisk eggs and sugar together. Slowly pour on milk, then pass through a sieve.

5 Flavour the milk with Grand Marnier, then pour the liquid over the bread and pears. Let it soak for 10 minutes so that bread absorbs the milk.

6 Place into oven 150°C, 300°F, Gas Mark 2 for 30-45 minutes or until you can put a knife into the centre and it comes out clean.

7 If you want, you can sprinkle the top of the pudding with sugar and glaze it under the grill until the sugar caramelises.

8 Serve with cream or custard flavoured with Grand Marnier.

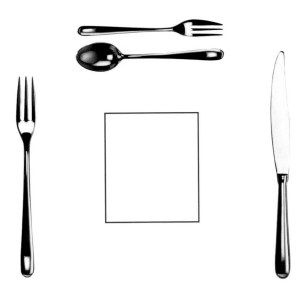

Starters	Kcal	kJ	Protein grams	Fat grams	Na mmol	K mmol	PO₄ mmol
Carrot & Coriander Soup	38	160	0.41	2.32	3.90	1.42	0.32
Onion & Rosemary Tart Tatin	343	1426	4.15	23.67	11.77	4.15	1.78
Cream of Courgette & Cumin Soup	30	126	1.24	1.17	1.61	5.22	0.72
Cream of Cauliflower & Mustard Soup	48	189	1.59	2.66	8.96	5.81	1.14
Chicken Spring Rolls	255	1228	10.94	16.18	7.05	5.85	3.71
Asian Spring Roll Dipping Sauce	68	291	0.11	0.02	0.02	0.53	0.07
Pan Fried Salmon with Ginger & Basil Sauce	731	3041	22.00	69.00	3.00	15.00	10.00

Main Courses

	Kcal	kJ	Protein grams	Fat grams	Na mmol	K mmol	PO₄ mmol
Thai Fish Cakes	123	516	15.33	6.80	15.22	8.44	5.92
Thai Cucumber Salad	33	142	0.72	0.10	0.47	3.40	1.22
Leek Turnovers	929	3860	10.10	73.36	54.49	11.69	5.65
Barbecued Tofu	467	1950	32.70	30.06	1.82	16.20	12.97
Peppered Tarragon Halibut with Carrot Puree	292	1218	30.00	19.00	6.00	12.00	10.00
Anise Carrot Puree	154	633	0.86	15.29	9.12	3.57	0.71
Five Spice Glazed Pork Chops	322	1350	39.70	16.24	4.73	18.58	12.79

	Kcal	kJ	Protein grams	Fat grams	Na mmol	K mmol	PO₄ mmol
Grilled Lamb with Couscous Salad	1349	5599	74.36	101.87	10.03	32.69	25.34
Polenta Terrine	103	425	1.20	6.70	5.03	0.94	0.05
Red Onion, Basil & Potato Salad	328	1369	3.25	21.00	6.00	12.00	2.00
Tarragon and Mustard Butter	213	876	0.48	23.36	11.82	0.46	0.48
Hollandaise Sauce	316	1300	2.12	33.80	12.72	1.78	2.38
Celeriac Gratin	74	304	0.65	7.26	2.45	3.42	0.80
White Cabbage with Cream Cheese	491	2023	4.13	49.19	16.38	11.19	0.37
Spiced Cod Mousse with Onion & Tomato Salad	378	1576	12.00	23.70	26.50	10.70	7.00
Saffron & Rosemary Crusted Chicken	500	2085	65.80	25.90	6.30	26.00	20.00
Saffron Risotto	573	2393	6.64	35.61	41.26	6.10	4.05
Crispy Grilled Lemon Sole	683	2835	26.17	54.89	8.00	10.00	10.00
Spiced Red Lentils	379	1590	16.16	17.67	12.48	22.00	8.60

Desserts

	Kcal	kJ	Protein grams	Fat grams	Na mmol	K mmol	PO₄ mmol
Lemon Tart	107	449	2.00	6.50	2.00	0.75	0.87
Jam Turnovers	357	1503	3.54	13.22	8.29	1.63	1.16
Lemon Meringue Pie	496	2086	5.74	20.31	11.29	2.34	2.54
Lemon Cream Cheese Pound Cake	916	3853	9.33	40.93	23.66	4.24	9.47
Devonshire Apple Cake	297	1242	3.46	16.51	9.86	5.87	1.80
Steamed Lemon Sponge Pudding	378	1580	5.92	23.15	5.45	5.81	4.43
Peach Crumble	385	1616	5.27	17.87	7.90	6.96	3.60
Glazed Rice Pudding	289	1218	8.77	10.21	5.46	8.17	7.62
Pear & Grand Marnier Bread & Butter Pudding	390	1639	10.41	17.07	14.31	7.54	6.43

Na   – **Sodium**
K   – **Potassium**
PO₄   – **Phosphorous**

USE FREELY	USE CAREFULLY	AVOID OR USE ONLY A PINCH
LOW POTASSIUM	MODERATE POTASSIUM	HIGH POTASSIUM
Cinnamon	Black Pepper	Dried Oregano
Nutmeg	Cayenne Pepper	Dried Basil
Sesame Seeds	Saffron	Coriander Leaves
Ginger Root	Dried Sage	Dried Parsley
Tamarind Leaves	Dried Marjoram	Dried Tarragon
Mustard	Dried Mint	Chilli Powder
Fresh Tarragon	Dried Cloves	Turmeric
White Pepper	Fresh Dill	Paprika
Fresh/Dried Rosemary	Fresh Parsley	Dried Dill
Fresh Mint	Fresh Oregano	Fennel Seeds
Garlic	Fresh Basil	
Vinegar	Chinese Five Spice	
Mint Sauce	Allspice	
	Mild Curry Powder	
	Caraway Seeds	
	Cardamom	
	Coriander Seeds	
	Cumin	
	Fresh Chilli	
	Garam Masala	
	Ginger Powder	
	Fenugreek Seeds	

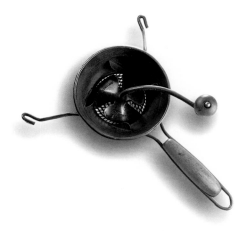

VEGETABLES
One Portion = 85g

USE IN MODERATION

USE CAREFULLY*

SALAD

CHOOSE FROM**

Asparagus	Brussel Sprouts	¹/₂ tomato or 2 cherry tomatoes
Aubergine	Fennel	2 slices of beetroot
Beansprouts	Mushrooms	1 stick of celery
Broccoli	Okra	5 slices of cucumber
Cabbage - all types	Parsnips	30g watercress
Carrots	Spinach	30g lettuce
Cauliflower		4 rings of peppers
Chicory		4 radishes
Courgette		3 spring onions
Green Beans		
Leek		
Mange Tout		
Marrow		
Mixed vegetables		
Onions		
Peas		
Pumpkin		
Runner Beans		
Spring Onion		
Swede		
Turnip		

IF ON A POTASSIUM RESTRICTED DIET:

- Avoid these vegetables*

- All vegetables should be boiled and the water discarded and not used for sauces or gravy.

- Two portions of vegetables are allowed daily (with each portion weighing no more than 85g).

- A portion of salad consists of TWO items from the list, and is exchanged for a portion of vegetables**

- A portion of potatoes is approximately 150g.

1

Starter	Carrot and Coriander Soup
Main Course	Grilled Lamb with Couscous Salad
Dessert	Lemon Tart

Total Nutritional Values

1494 Kcal	6208 kJ	76.77g Protein	110.69g Fat
15.93 mmol Na	34.86 mmol K	26.53 mmol PO_4	

2

Starter	Onion and Rosemary Tart Tatin
Main Course	Peppered Tarragon Halibut with Carrot Puree
Dessert	Steamed Lemon Sponge

Total Nutritional Values

1013 Kcal	4224 kJ	40.07g Protein	65.82g Fat
23.22 mmol Na	21.96 mmol K	16.21 mmol PO_4	

Excludes vegetables. If a portion of potatoes and two low potassium vegetable are eaten this will increase the total potassium by approximately 15-20 mmol.

WEIGHTS

15g	$\frac{1}{2}$ oz
28g	1 oz
55g	2 oz
85g	3 oz
100g	3 $\frac{1}{2}$ oz
110g	4 oz
140g	5 oz
170g	6 oz
200g	7 oz
225g	8 oz
255g	9 oz
285g	10 oz
310g	11 oz
340g	12 oz
370g	13 oz
400g	14 oz
425g	15 oz
450g	1 lb
500g	1 lb 2 oz
570g	1 $\frac{1}{4}$ lb
680g	1 $\frac{1}{2}$ lb
900g	2 lb
1kg	2 lb 3 oz

LIQUID MEASURES

5ml	1 teaspoon (tsp)	
15ml	1 tablespoon (tbsp)	
120ml	4 floz	
150ml	5 floz	$\frac{1}{4}$ pint
175ml	6 floz	
200ml	7 floz	$\frac{1}{3}$ pint
250ml	8 floz	
300ml	10 floz	$\frac{1}{2}$ pint
350ml	12 floz	
400ml	14 floz	
450ml	15 floz	$\frac{3}{4}$ pint
500 ml	18 floz	
600ml	20 floz	1 pint
750ml		1 $\frac{1}{4}$ pints
900ml		1 $\frac{1}{2}$ pints
1 litre		1 $\frac{3}{4}$ pints

These measurements are approximate conversions only, which we have rounded up or down. It is important not to mix metric and imperial measures in one recipe.

DIMENSIONS OF CUTTERS

2.5 cm	1 inch
5 cm	2 inches
10 cm	4 inches
18 cm	7 inches
20 cm	8 inches
23 cm	9 inches

OVEN TEMPERATURES

very cool	- 110°C/225°F gas mark $\frac{1}{4}$
	- 120°C/250°F gas mark $\frac{1}{2}$
cool	- 140°C/250°F gas mark 1
	- 150°C/300°F gas mark 2
moderate	- 160°C/325°F gas mark 3
	- 180°C/350°F gas mark 4
moderately hot	- 190°C/375°F gas mark 5
	- 200°C/400°F gas mark 6
hot	- 220°C/425°F gas mark 7
	- 230°C/450°F gas mark 8
very hot	- 240°C/475°F gas mark 9

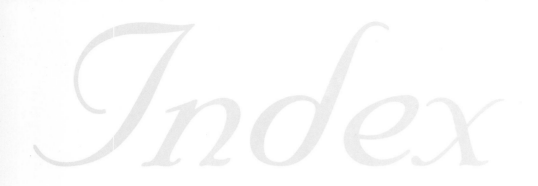